Medicinal Herbs
25 Useful Healing Herbs To Use, Grow, And Dry

Table of content

Introduction

You wander the shelves at the store, looking over row after row of different and supplements and pills for a variety of ailments. You are supposed to take pill after pill and remedy any situation with one pill after another.

No matter what the issue is, where the problem is, or what you are doing with your life, you have to take a pill for this reason, for that reason, or for any other reason. No matter what the reason, this is the solution for everyone.

But that is not the way it is supposed to be.

We are designed to heal naturally, and we are supposed to use the natural world around us to remain our best selves. With this in mind, you are forced to turn to synthetic after synthetic, and wonder if you are really doing yourself any good with what you are putting in your body.

But that doesn't have to be the case.

You can grow, cultivate, and preserve your very own herbal remedies, and never have to worry about your health again. No matter what your health goals are, you are going to find the exact same results in the herbs that you grow as you would out of the pills that you purchase.

"But I have never grown my own herbs, what do I do?"

"Are preserving herbs difficult? I want to grow some, but I want to save them, too. How can I make both of this happen?"

"Is this hard? I want to grow herbs, but I don't have a green thumb, and the last thing I need is for the herbs to wither and die."

If you haven't grown herbs yourself before, odds are you are wondering how to grow them and keep them. Now, you don't have to. This book is going to show you exactly what you need to do to grow your own herbs, care for them, and preserve them for the greatest use.

Whether you have never grown your own herbs before, or if you are a seasoned grower, you are going to learn exactly what you need in this book.

So if you are ready to grow your own little garden of health, you have come to the right place. Jump on in.

Chapter 1 – The Green Things

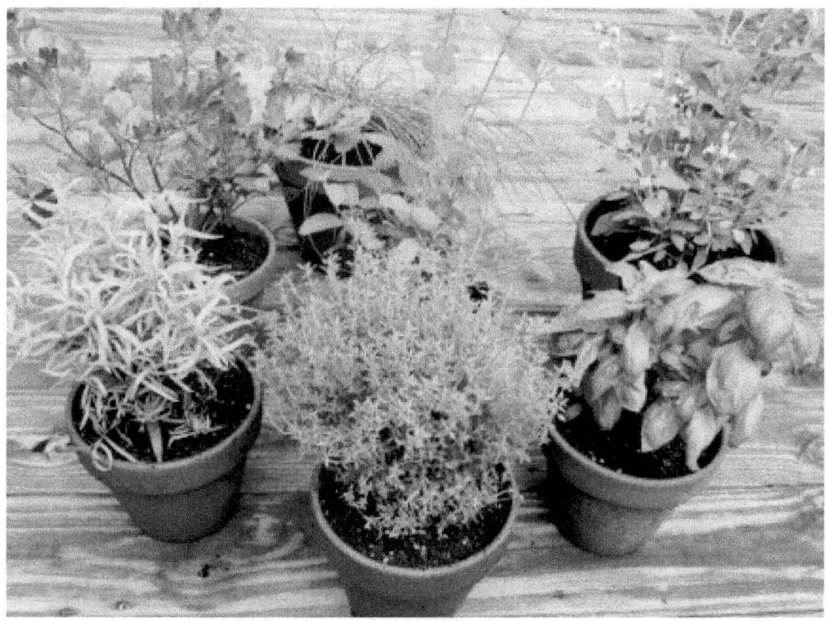

Lavender

How to grow

Lavender is easy to grow, and will work in many climates. Simply choose the variety that you like best, and plant in a pot. Store the pot in a sunny area and water often.

How to harvest and preserve

Simply grow your plant until they are mature. You will be able to see that they are by the way the leaves grow.

When they are fully developed and a uniform color, they are ready. Simply take your gardening scissors and snip off the leaves right at the base where they grow onto the stem.

Make sure you do not harm the stem as you work.

Lay them out on a paper towel to dry, or speed the process in a food dehydrator. When they are completely dried out, scoop the leaves into a small glass jar with an airtight lid until you are ready to use them.

Uses:

Perfect to add the sweet kick to desserts and teas, relaxing.

Licorice

How to grow

Soak the seeds for 24 hours before planting them at a depth of ½ inch. Water often.

How to harvest and preserve

Simply grow your plant until they are mature. You will be able to see that they are by the way the leaves grow.

When they are fully developed and a uniform color, they are ready. Simply take your gardening scissors and snip off the leaves right at the base where they grow onto the stem.

Make sure you do not harm the stem as you work.

Lay them out on a paper towel to dry, or speed the process in a food dehydrator. When they are completely dried out, scoop the leaves into a small glass jar with an airtight lid until you are ready to use them.

Uses:

An incredible flavoring agent, perfect for anti-inflammatory use.

Marshmallow

How to grow

Soak the seeds for 24 hours before planting them. Water infrequently, keeping the water moist but not too wet.

How to harvest and preserve

Simply grow your plant until they are mature. You will be able to see that they are by the way the leaves grow.

When they are fully developed and a uniform color, they are ready. Simply take your gardening scissors and snip off the leaves right at the base where they grow onto the stem.

Make sure you do not harm the stem as you work.

Lay them out on a paper towel to dry, or speed the process in a food dehydrator. When they are completely dried out, scoop the leaves into a small glass jar with an airtight lid until you are ready to use them.

Uses:

The perfect go-to herb for dry or flaky skin, use this to soothe even the driest of hands.

Rosemary

How to grow

One of the easiest to grow herbs, use simply plant a few seeds in a pot and water lightly.

How to harvest and preserve

Simply grow your plant until they are mature. You will be able to see that they are by the way the leaves grow.

When they are fully developed and a uniform color, they are ready. Simply take your gardening scissors and snip off the leaves right at the base where they grow onto the stem.

Make sure you do not harm the stem as you work.

Lay them out on a paper towel to dry, or speed the process in a food dehydrator. When they are completely dried out, scoop the leaves into a small glass jar with an airtight lid until you are ready to use them.

Uses:

Excellent for cooking, this incredible herb shows signs of preventing cancer and fighting illness.

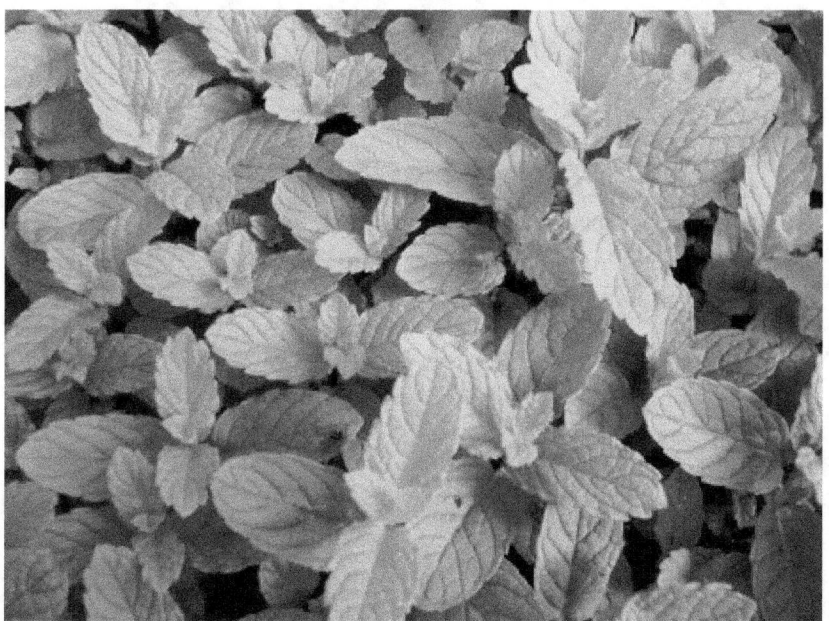

Thyme

How to grow

Thyme, much like rosemary, is incredibly easy to grow. Simply plant a few seeds in some soil and leave in the sun, watering often but not too frequently.

How to harvest and preserve

Simply grow your plant until they are mature. You will be able to see that they are by the way the leaves grow.

When they are fully developed and a uniform color, they are ready. Simply take your gardening scissors and snip off the leaves right at the base where they grow onto the stem.

Make sure you do not harm the stem as you work.

Lay them out on a paper towel to dry, or speed the process in a food dehydrator. When they are completely dried out, scoop the leaves into a small glass jar with an airtight lid until you are ready to use them.

Uses:

Thyme is the best herb to turn to for bronchitis and other respiratory ailments. Keep some on hand for any number of issues that could arise, even sore throats.

Chapter 2 – Perfect Plants for Any Plans

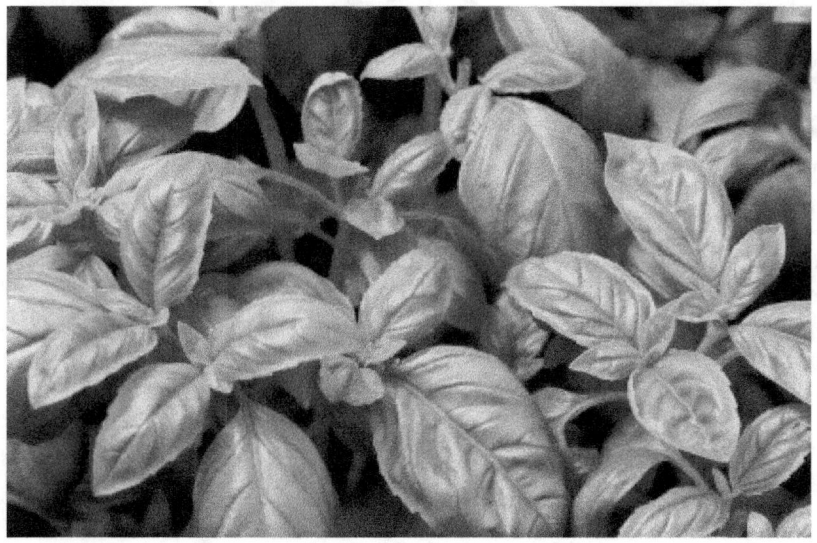

Lemon Balm

How to grow

Plant seeds sparingly in a pot, and keep in direct sunlight. Water morning and evening.

How to harvest and preserve

Simply grow your plant until they are mature. You will be able to see that they are by the way the leaves grow.

When they are fully developed and a uniform color, they are ready. Simply take your gardening scissors and snip off the leaves right at the base where they grow onto the stem.

Make sure you do not harm the stem as you work.

Lay them out on a paper towel to dry, or speed the process in a food dehydrator. When they are completely dried out, scoop the leaves into a small glass jar with an airtight lid until you are ready to use them.

Uses:

This plant has incredible calming effects. Use it to relax, calm anxiety, and soothe any fears.

Lemon Verbena

How to grow

Plant seeds sparingly in a pot, and keep in direct sunlight. Water morning and evening.

How to harvest and preserve

Simply grow your plant until they are mature. You will be able to see that they are by the way the leaves grow.

When they are fully developed and a uniform color, they are ready. Simply take your gardening scissors and snip off the leaves right at the base where they grow onto the stem.

Make sure you do not harm the stem as you work.

Lay them out on a paper towel to dry, or speed the process in a food dehydrator. When they are completely dried out, scoop the leaves into a small glass jar with an airtight lid until you are ready to use them.

Uses:

This is the plant to turn to if you are looking to lose weight and feel great. Anti inflammatory properties also make this a prime choice for swollen joints and pain.

Fennel

How to grow

Plant seeds sparingly in a pot, and keep in direct sunlight. Water morning and evening.

How to harvest and preserve

Simply grow your plant until they are mature. You will be able to see that they are by the way the leaves grow.

When they are fully developed and a uniform color, they are ready. Simply take your gardening scissors and snip off the leaves right at the base where they grow onto the stem.

Make sure you do not harm the stem as you work.

Lay them out on a paper towel to dry, or speed the process in a food dehydrator. When they are completely dried out, scoop the leaves into a small glass jar with an airtight lid until you are ready to use them.

Uses:

A member of the carrot family, this is a great herb to use for weight loss, healthy eyesight, and immunity.

Saint John's Wort

How to grow

Plant seeds sparingly in a pot, and keep in direct sunlight. Water morning and evening.

How to harvest and preserve

Simply grow your plant until they are mature. You will be able to see that they are by the way the leaves grow.

When they are fully developed and a uniform color, they are ready. Simply take your gardening scissors and snip off the leaves right at the base where they grow onto the stem.

Make sure you do not harm the stem as you work.

Lay them out on a paper towel to dry, or speed the process in a food dehydrator. When they are completely dried out, scoop the leaves into a small glass jar with an airtight lid until you are ready to use them.

Uses:

This could be considered the 'good mood' herb. Many people use Saint John's Wort as a natural form of an anti-depressant.

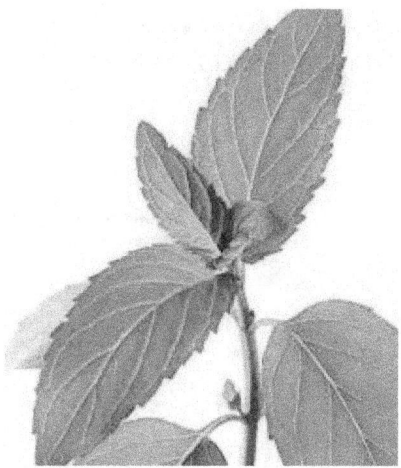

Basil

How to grow

Plant seeds sparingly in a pot, and keep in direct sunlight. Water morning and evening.

How to harvest and preserve

Simply grow your plant until they are mature. You will be able to see that they are by the way the leaves grow.

When they are fully developed and a uniform color, they are ready. Simply take your gardening scissors and snip off the leaves right at the base where they grow onto the stem.

Make sure you do not harm the stem as you work.

Lay them out on a paper towel to dry, or speed the process in a food dehydrator. When they are completely dried out, scoop the leaves into a small glass jar with an airtight lid until you are ready to use them.

Uses:

Though this is an herb that is rich in flavor and can be used for a variety of health benefits including anti-inflammatory.

Chapter 3 – From the Garden to the Table

Parsley

How to grow

Section plants roughly 1 inch apart in your pot, and place in a sunny area. Water daily.

How to harvest and preserve

Simply grow your plant until they are mature. You will be able to see that they are by the way the leaves grow.

When they are fully developed and a uniform color, they are ready. Simply take your gardening scissors and snip off the leaves right at the base where they grow onto the stem.

Make sure you do not harm the stem as you work.

Lay them out on a paper towel to dry, or speed the process in a food dehydrator. When they are completely dried out, scoop the leaves into a small glass jar with an airtight lid until you are ready to use them.

Uses:

Full of antioxidants, this is the perfect herb to use for all over health. By using this herb frequently, you are going to have an overall feeling of health and wellness.

Parsley is an excellent source of folic acid, meaning it is one of the best things you can consume for your heart. Not only that, but it is another excellent herb to include in your diet if you want to lose weight.

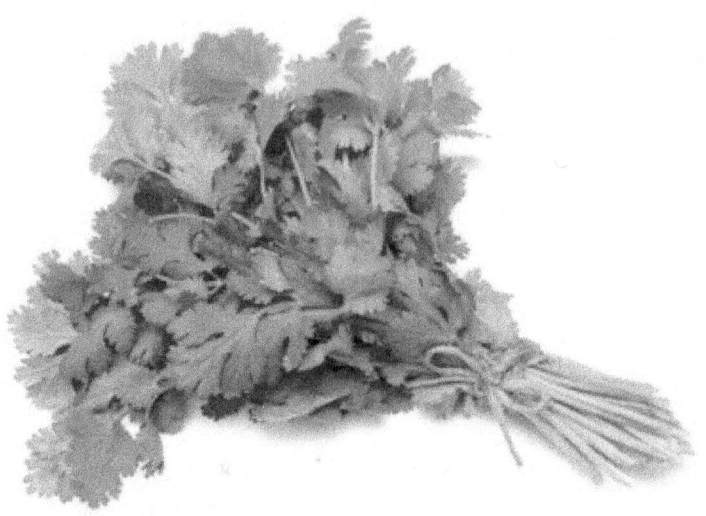

Cilantro

How to grow

Section plants roughly 1 inch apart in your pot, and place in a sunny area. Water daily.

How to harvest and preserve

Simply grow your plant until they are mature. You will be able to see that they are by the way the leaves grow.

When they are fully developed and a uniform color, they are ready. Simply take your gardening scissors and snip off the leaves right at the base where they grow onto the stem.

Make sure you do not harm the stem as you work.

Lay them out on a paper towel to dry, or speed the process in a food dehydrator. When they are completely dried out, scoop the leaves into a small glass jar with an airtight lid until you are ready to use them.

Uses:

Choose this herb for all of your cholesterol needs, and be ready to embrace the antioxidants that run abundantly through the leaves. This is the herb to turn to for excellent blood health.

Oregano

How to grow

Section plants roughly 1 inch apart in your pot, and place in a sunny area. Water daily.

How to harvest and preserve

Simply grow your plant until they are mature. You will be able to see that they are by the way the leaves grow.

When they are fully developed and a uniform color, they are ready. Simply take your gardening scissors and snip off the leaves right at the base where they grow onto the stem.

Make sure you do not harm the stem as you work.

Lay them out on a paper towel to dry, or speed the process in a food dehydrator. When they are completely dried out, scoop the leaves into a small glass jar with an airtight lid until you are ready to use them.

Uses:

This is a plant that is rich in vitamin K. Potassium and antioxidants are also found here, making this not only a great herb to cook with for the taste, but one you should choose for the health benefits as well.

Chives

How to grow

Section plants roughly 1 inch apart in your pot, and place in a sunny area. Water daily.

How to harvest and preserve

Simply grow your plant until they are mature. You will be able to see that they are by the way the leaves grow.

When they are fully developed and a uniform color, they are ready. Simply take your gardening scissors and snip off the leaves right at the base where they grow onto the stem.

Make sure you do not harm the stem as you work.

Lay them out on a paper towel to dry, or speed the process in a food dehydrator. When they are completely dried out, scoop the leaves into a small glass jar with an airtight lid until you are ready to use them.

Uses:

I could spend an entire day explaining all of the excellent benefits of chives. They are great for your circulatory system perhaps most importantly, and they are rich in vitamins.

Include in your diet often for maximum results.

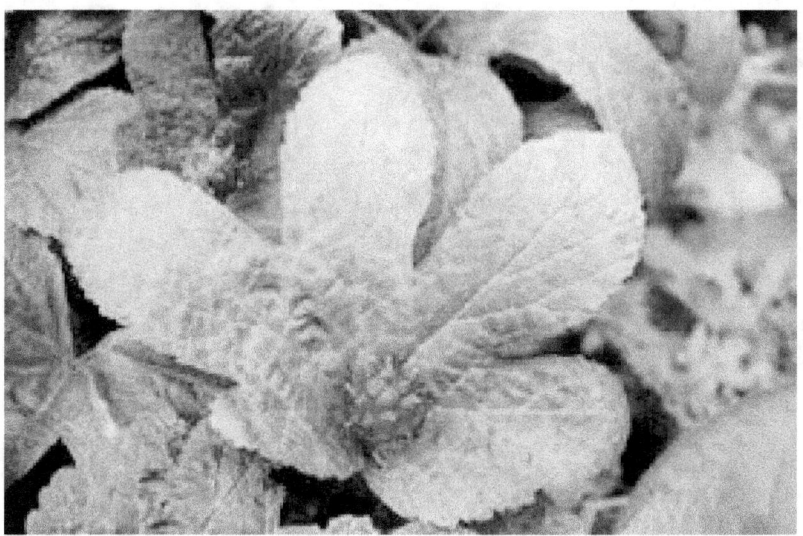

Goldenseal

How to grow

Section plants roughly 1 inch apart in your pot, and place in a sunny area. Water daily.

How to harvest and preserve

Simply grow your plant until they are mature. You will be able to see that they are by the way the leaves grow.

When they are fully developed and a uniform color, they are ready. Simply take your gardening scissors and snip off the leaves right at the base where they grow onto the stem.

Make sure you do not harm the stem as you work.

Lay them out on a paper towel to dry, or speed the process in a food dehydrator. When they are completely dried out, scoop the leaves into a small glass jar with an airtight lid until you are ready to use them.

Uses:

In this modern world we live in, I can't say enough good things about a plant that fights cancer, and not only does this plant help prevent cancer cells from forming, it is also effective in fighting the illness.

Chapter 4 – Minty Madness

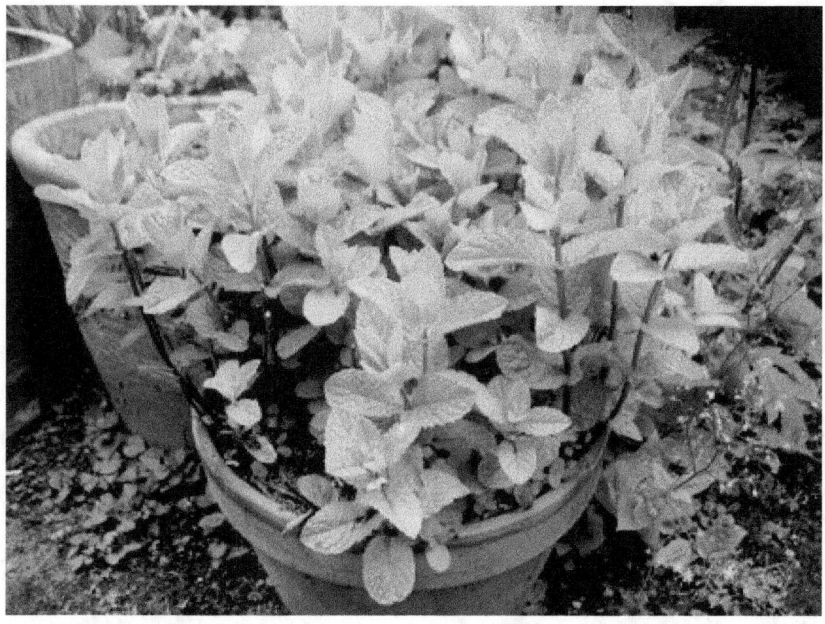

Peppermint

How to grow

Mints in general are really easy to grow. Place in a pot and leave in direct sunlight, water daily.

How to harvest and preserve

Simply grow your plant until they are mature. You will be able to see that they are by the way the leaves grow.

When they are fully developed and a uniform color, they are ready. Simply take your gardening scissors and snip off the leaves right at the base where they grow onto the stem.

Make sure you do not harm the stem as you work.

Lay them out on a paper towel to dry, or speed the process in a food dehydrator. When they are completely dried out, scoop the leaves into a small glass jar with an airtight lid until you are ready to use them.

Uses:

A wide array of uses come with this lovely mint. Use for aches and sores, headaches, stomach aches, or any other joint pain.

Spearmint

How to grow

Place in a pot and leave in direct sunlight, water daily.

How to harvest and preserve

Simply grow your plant until they are mature. You will be able to see that they are by the way the leaves grow.

When they are fully developed and a uniform color, they are ready. Simply take your gardening scissors and snip off the leaves right at the base where they grow onto the stem.

Make sure you do not harm the stem as you work.

Lay them out on a paper towel to dry, or speed the process in a food dehydrator. When they are completely dried out, scoop the leaves into a small glass jar with an airtight lid until you are ready to use them.

Uses:

Use to flavor meats and savory dishes, teas, and medicinally for aches and pains.

Lemon Mint

How to grow

Place in a pot and leave in direct sunlight, water daily.

How to harvest and preserve

Simply grow your plant until they are mature. You will be able to see that they are by the way the leaves grow.

When they are fully developed and a uniform color, they are ready. Simply take your gardening scissors and snip off the leaves right at the base where they grow onto the stem.

Make sure you do not harm the stem as you work.

Lay them out on a paper towel to dry, or speed the process in a food dehydrator. When they are completely dried out, scoop the leaves into a small glass jar with an airtight lid until you are ready to use them.

Uses:

Use to flavor meats and savory dishes, teas, and medicinally for aches and pains.

Apple Mint

How to grow

Place in a pot and leave in direct sunlight, water daily.

How to harvest and preserve

Simply grow your plant until they are mature. You will be able to see that they are by the way the leaves grow.

When they are fully developed and a uniform color, they are ready. Simply take your gardening scissors and snip off the leaves right at the base where they grow onto the stem.

Make sure you do not harm the stem as you work.

Lay them out on a paper towel to dry, or speed the process in a food dehydrator. When they are completely dried out, scoop the leaves into a small glass jar with an airtight lid until you are ready to use them.

Uses:

Use to flavor meats and savory dishes, teas, and medicinally for aches and pains.

Chocolate Mint

How to grow

Place in a pot and leave in direct sunlight, water daily.

How to harvest and preserve

Simply grow your plant until they are mature. You will be able to see that they are by the way the leaves grow.

When they are fully developed and a uniform color, they are ready. Simply take your gardening scissors and snip off the leaves right at the base where they grow onto the stem.

Make sure you do not harm the stem as you work.

Lay them out on a paper towel to dry, or speed the process in a food dehydrator. When they are completely dried out, scoop the leaves into a small glass jar with an airtight lid until you are ready to use them.

Uses:

Use to flavor meats and savory dishes, teas, and medicinally for aches and pains.

Chapter 5 – The Best of the Rest

Tarragon

How to grow

Plant seeds roughly ½ inch into the soil, and space them 1 inch apart. Set in a well lit area and water frequently.

How to harvest and preserve

Simply grow your plant until they are mature. You will be able to see that they are by the way the leaves grow.

When they are fully developed and a uniform color, they are ready. Simply take your gardening scissors and snip off the leaves right at the base where they grow onto the stem.

Make sure you do not harm the stem as you work.

Lay them out on a paper towel to dry, or speed the process in a food dehydrator. When they are completely dried out, scoop the leaves into a small glass jar with an airtight lid until you are ready to use them.

Uses:

Another essential herb for your blood. This is the herb to turn to for heart health. You will find that it lowers your blood pressure, evens out your blood sugar, and it helps prevent blood clots.

An all in one herb for perfection.

Sage

How to grow

Plant seeds roughly ½ inch into the soil, and space them 1 inch apart. Set in a well lit area and water frequently.

How to harvest and preserve

Simply grow your plant until they are mature. You will be able to see that they are by the way the leaves grow.

When they are fully developed and a uniform color, they are ready. Simply take your gardening scissors and snip off the leaves right at the base where they grow onto the stem.

Make sure you do not harm the stem as you work.

Lay them out on a paper towel to dry, or speed the process in a food dehydrator. When they are completely dried out, scoop the leaves into a small glass jar with an airtight lid until you are ready to use them.

Uses:

Sage is excellent for the digestive tract. Take it and promote a healthy gut.

Marigold

How to grow

Plant seeds roughly ½ inch into the soil, and space them 1 inch apart. Set in a well lit area and water frequently.

How to harvest and preserve

Simply grow your plant until they are mature. You will be able to see that they are by the way the leaves grow.

When they are fully developed and a uniform color, they are ready. Simply take your gardening scissors and snip off the leaves right at the base where they grow onto the stem.

Make sure you do not harm the stem as you work.

Lay them out on a paper towel to dry, or speed the process in a food dehydrator. When they are completely dried out, scoop the leaves into a small glass jar with an airtight lid until you are ready to use them.

Uses:

Marigold has been used as an anti-inflammatory as well as a relief for stomach pain. Keep it on hand for a variety of ailments.

Feverfew

How to grow

Plant seeds roughly ½ inch into the soil, and space them 1 inch apart. Set in a well lit area and water frequently.

How to harvest and preserve

Simply grow your plant until they are mature. You will be able to see that they are by the way the leaves grow.

When they are fully developed and a uniform color, they are ready. Simply take your gardening scissors and snip off the leaves right at the base where they grow onto the stem.

Make sure you do not harm the stem as you work.

Lay them out on a paper towel to dry, or speed the process in a food dehydrator. When they are completely dried out, scoop the leaves into a small glass jar with an airtight lid until you are ready to use them.

Uses:

An herb used to treat headaches and joint pain, this is the herb to have on hand if you work with your hands often. It is going to ease a lot of the pain without all of the side effects of synthetic medication.

Chamomile

How to grow

Plant seeds roughly ½ inch into the soil, and space them 1 inch apart. Set in a well lit area and water frequently.

How to harvest and preserve

Simply grow your plant until they are mature. You will be able to see that they are by the way the leaves grow.

When they are fully developed and a uniform color, they are ready. Simply take your gardening scissors and snip off the leaves right at the base where they grow onto the stem.

Make sure you do not harm the stem as you work.

Lay them out on a paper towel to dry, or speed the process in a food dehydrator. When they are completely dried out, scoop the leaves into a small glass jar with an airtight lid until you are ready to use them.

Uses:

Welcome relaxation into your life when you indulge in this rich herb. Perfect to chill out even the most stressful day.

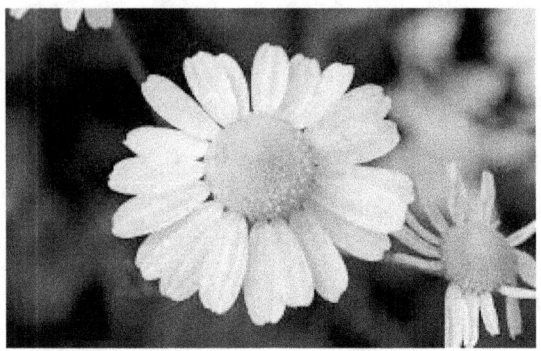

Conclusion

There you have it, everything you need to know to grow your own herbs, preserve your own herbs, and make them exactly what you need them to be. I know there are a lot of different things you can read online about growing and keeping your own plants, but the fact of the matter is that you can do it quickly and easily.

This book is going to show you exactly what you need to do to grow your own herbs, and what you need to do to get the most out of them, no matter what you need to use them for. I want you to be successful in your herbs, and I want you to see the real methods you can use to reap the benefits.

I know there is a lot of excitement when you are beginning this project, and I hope you don't lose any of that enthusiasm. This book is going to show you anything and everything you need to grow and use your own herbs.

Remember that if you don't get what you want the first time around, then stick with it. There are times when you need work at things before you get the results that you want. There's nothing wrong with trying something more than once before you get the results that you are after, and there's no shame in doing things different ways to find the method that works for you.

I have designed this book to be exactly what you need to get started in your new endeavor, and with practice, you are going to get the exact herb garden you have always wanted.

So if you are ready to take a step back from all of those synthetic medications you have seen on the shelves of the store, and if you are ready to jump into the world of herbal remedies, you need look no further than this book.

You are going to get everything you have ever wanted in herbs, and this book is going to be with your every step of the way. Are you ready to let your inner gardener out?

Roll up your sleeves and slip on your gloves.

The garden awaits.

FREE Bonus Reminder

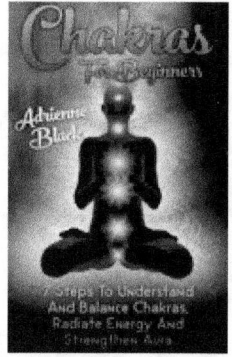

If you have not grabbed it yet, please go ahead and download your special bonus E book *"Chakras for Beginners. 7 Steps To Understand And Balance Chakras, Radiate Energy, And Strengthen Aura"*.

Simply Click the Button Below

Click Here to
Download the ebook

OR Go to This Page

http://lifehacksworld.com/free

BONUS #2: More Free & Discounted Books & Products

Do you want to receive more Free/Discounted Books or Products?

We have a mailing list where we send out our new Books or Products when they go free or with a discount on Amazon. Click on the link below to sign up for Free & Discount Book & Product Promotions.

=> Sign Up for Free & Discount Book & Product Promotions <=

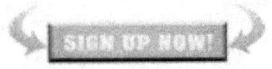

OR Go to this URL

http://zbit.ly/1WBb1Ek